Influenza Pandemic Response Plan for Office Buildings

Taking Action during an Influenza Pandemic

Karen J. Bates

iUniverse, Inc.
Bloomington

Influenza Pandemic Response Plan for Office Buildings
Taking Action during an Influenza Pandemic

iUniverse books may be ordered through booksellers or by contacting:

iUniverse
1663 Liberty Drive
Bloomington, IN 47403
www.iuniverse.com
1-800-Authors (1-800-288-4677)

ISBN: 978-1-4620-1162-9 (sc)
ISBN: 978-1-4620-1163-6 (e)

Printed in the United States of America

iUniverse rev. date: 07/07/2011

Acknowledgment

I wish to acknowledge Tiffin Bak, a loyal employee who worked for me for many years and still wishes to be my friend. Without her assistance and perseverance, this manual would not have been possible.

Disclaimer

The material and information in this manual is intended solely as a guide and not a complete source of information or plan for the reader's particular office building during or after an influenza pandemic. Every building is unique and requires specific planning with the assistance of a professional. This writer makes no warranties or representations, express or implied, regarding the information in this manual or its use by the reader. All charts, graphs, and any other forms printed in this manual were created and designed solely by this writer; any similarities to other forms are strictly coincidental. By accepting and reading this manual, the reader acknowledges that the writer is not responsible for the completeness, keeping the information current, or its use on any other basis by the reader. The reader does, hereby, waive any and all claims against the writer arising out of reader's use or reliance of this manual.

Contents

Managing Agent Guidelines

Tenant Responsibilities

Practice Drills

Post-Influenza Pandemic

Appendix

Glossary of Terms

The following terms will help you as you navigate through this manual.

Alert levels are based upon information received from local, state, and federal health organizations.

Cross-Training is used throughout this manual to describe employees learning more than one task to operate the building effectively. It can also be used to learn another employee's duties. This protects the building when regular personnel are not able to perform their normal duties.

The **decision team** is a group of people within the building composed of the property manager, head of building maintenance, head of building operations, security supervisor, cleaning area manager, and any other key individuals that would add to the specific situation. The size of this decision team would also be determined by the size of the building and the composition of personnel.

Large groups are defined as being ten or more people.

HVAC is an acronym for heating, ventilating, and air-conditioning.

Mission-critical is used to describe something that is of primary importance in the process. This terminology is used in the "Building Maintenance Guidelines" section of this manual.

The **World Health Organization (WHO)** uses a six-phased approach for easy incorporation of new recommendations and approaches into existing national preparedness and response plans. For detailed information and current alert status, go to their website at **www.who.int** and look for avian influenza data in the section titled "Global Alert and Response (GAR)."

Influenza Pandemic Readiness Summaries

(These alert levels are based upon information received from local, state, and federal health organizations.)

	Alert Level 1	Alert Level 2	Alert Level 3
Description	Outside of North America (pandemic not yet declared)	Outbreaks have spread to North America	First case in United States
Building Management Action	1. Issue communication to tenants about influenza pandemic 2. Order raw materials 3. Begin build of inventory 4. Acquire safety supplies 5. Cross-train personnel.	1. Build inventory 2. Ensure vendors have 3 mo. stock 3. Institute Decision Team process 4. Cross-train personnel 5. Update contact/ vendors lists 6. Ensure cleaning company and security have cross-trained their personnel	1. Continue to cross-train 2. Distribute safety supplies 3. Communicate policies
Decision Team Actions	No action necessary until alert level 5	No action necessary until alert level 5	No action necessary until alert level 5

	Alert Level 4	**Alert Level 5**	**Alert Level 6**
Description	First case in your state	First case in your area	First case in your building
Building Management Action	1. Increase cleaning protocols 2. Management fears 3. Execute plans 4. Increase cleaning inventory to six-month supply	1. Increase cleaning protocols 2. Restrict access to the building 3. Consult local government for assistance	1. Place building in off-hours mode. 2. Quarantine where necessary, including building staff
Decision Team Actions	No action necessary until alert level 5	1. Issues communication to tenants on family preparedness 2. Communicates critical functions to those responsible 3. Meets monthly	1. Meets weekly 2. Practices scenarios 3. Critical function practices

Preface

The *Influenza Pandemic Response Plan for Office Buildings* has been established as an operational guideline for building services designed to respond to a variety of emergency pandemic situations. However, there may be times when it has not addressed a specific situation.

Following the procedures in this manual will not assure or guarantee the safety of persons or property in the event of an influenza pandemic. It is intended to protect the building and its occupants with the utmost of care and to the best of its ability. It has also been designed to address situations when a specific person in charge is not able to carry out his or her duties.

Overall Objectives

Secure the Building

As the alert levels heighten, additional security and safety measures are essential for protection of personnel and the continuity of the workplace environment. Alert levels are escalated upon information received from local, state, and federal health organizations.

Enforcement of Hygiene Procedures

The possibility of an influenza pandemic is a concern to everyone. Although individuals cannot completely limit their exposure to the virus that causes influenza, there are things people can do to reduce the likelihood of becoming infected. This manual will encourage and promote good hygiene.

Control Air Flow throughout the Building

One major source of spreading influenza is through the building's heating and air-conditioning system. Building personnel need to define which building systems are mission-critical, examine the intake and exhaust systems, and determine how each system will treat the air and filtration process throughout the alert levels.

Maintain Building Personnel

The most critical aspect of any influenza pandemic is retaining building personnel who are familiar with the building and its operations. The number of man hours and skills needed to support the operations will be determined by the severity of the influenza pandemic.

Crisis Hotlines and Key Contacts

Crisis Hotline Telephone Numbers

City Health Department: _____

USA Department of Health and Human Services: 877-696-6775

Serious and life-threatening injuries: 911

Hospitals in the area: _____

Center for Disease Control and Prevention: 800-232-4636

Building Maintenance and Management Emergency Telephone Numbers

List all important building staff and management, including their home telephone, cell, and pager numbers where applicable. Include those designated as cross-trained. Be sure to list these contacts in their order of priority. See the sample chart below. It is very important to update this list on a quarterly basis.

Title	Name	Home Phone	Cell Phone	Pager
Property Manager				
Building Manager				
Operations Manager				
Lead Maintenance				
Building Maintenance – Cross-Trained				

Title	Name	Home Phone	Cell Phone	Pager
Building Maintenance – Cross-Trained				

Vendor Emergency Telephone Numbers

Vendor emergency telephone numbers are also important within your specific building. You will need to adapt the specific vendor list in relation to the type of property that you are operating. There can be more than one appropriate contact for a vendor depending upon the scope of services they provide. See the sample chart below. It is very important to update this list on a quarterly basis.

Company	Contact Name	Office Phone	Cell Phone	Pager
Security				
Elevator				
Cleaning				
HVAC				
Electric				
Gas				
Water & Sewer				

Paper Suppliers (list at least three companies
with office, cell, and e-mail addresses)

Cleaning Product Suppliers (list at least three
companies with office, cell, and e-mail addresses)

Cleaning Guidelines

Ongoing Personnel Training

As the threat of an influenza pandemic increases, it is imperative that the building carry out the proper cleaning and disinfecting procedures. This includes cross-training of building personnel to help minimize disruption and ensure continued service. In the event that the building uses an outside cleaning contractor, make sure your contract covers cross-training of its personnel. Also verify that they have an influenza pandemic response plan in place to ensure they are able to provide contracted services.

The labor pool can be greatly reduced due to transportation, employee demographics, and level of panic in the community. Therefore it is critical to have cleaners trained in the building specifications who live within a short distance.

- Post a written job description in the supervisor's office of each cleaning personnel's responsibilities relating to their respective floors during normal operation.

- Inform all cleaning personnel that there will be no hand shaking or other physical contact with another person. They should use their arm to cover any coughing or sneezing, and they should avoid touching their eyes, nose, and mouth.

- Spell out the specific cleaning supplies that will be used by cleaning personnel through each alert level of influenza pandemic. All disinfectants must list flu and virus claims on their labels.

- Ensure each cleaning employee is familiar with protective dust masks and disposable latex or nitril gloves. Ensure that they *always* wash their hands.

- The supervisor will keep an up-to-date listing in the building office of every cleaning employee working in the building, along with those who are cross-trained. This listing will include their addresses, proximity to the building, and emergency telephone numbers.

Stocking Cleaning Supplies

Alert Level 1—The building acts in a normal operational mode. Cleaning will be performed as normally contracted, including the scheduled number of cleaners.

Alert Level 2—The cleaning company will start building a three-month inventory of disinfectant cleaning solutions for all hard surfaces, door handles, dispensers, sinks, commodes, stairwell railings, drinking fountains, and anything else that would come in contact with hands. All disinfectants must list flu and virus claims on the labels.

Alert Level 3 –Continue building the inventory of required cleaning solutions.

Alert Level 4—The cleaning company will increase the inventory of disinfectant cleaning solutions to a six-month supply. Management will add a day porter or matron depending upon the size of the building and define his/her duties.

Alert Level 5 – No additional action necessary.

Alert Level 6—The type and amount of cleaning will be determined by the management and approved by the owner of the building. The need for cleaning supplies will be established from this determination. Add one additional day porter or matron as needed.

Cleaning at Different Levels of an Influenza Pandemic

Coverage and cleaning frequency will be established by management and approved by the owner given the level of the influenza pandemic and the unique circumstances within the building. Normally scheduled cleaning may be adjusted based upon these circumstances. Special attention must be given during the disinfection process so that the proper dwell times for all disinfectants are permitted, to maximize disinfection. A cleaning frequency checklist is recommended, especially during alert levels 4–6. A sample checklist can be found in the appendix entitled "Cleaning Schedule Guidelines."

Alert Levels 1-3—The building acts in a normal operational mode. Cleaning will be performed as normally contracted, including the number of cleaners.

Alert Level 4—The building implements the use of hand sanitizers by all building personnel, security officers, and cleaning personnel. All cleaning employees will wear disposable latex gloves; a special bin will be placed in a convenient and secured area for glove disposal. Cleaners will change floor mops, all rags, and other supplies daily prior to performing the following:

- Wash down with cleaning solution daily all elevator call buttons and hand rails within the elevator cabs, as well as the call buttons on each floor.

- Wipe all hard surfaces, such as desks and file cabinets, with EPA disinfectant cleaning solution. Use spray disinfectant on telephones daily.

- Wipe with disinfectant cleaning solution the handles on both sides of all doors throughout the building, including all exterior entrance door handles, every Monday, Wednesday, and Friday.

- Clean all light switches and thermostats throughout the building every Monday, Wednesday, and Friday.

- Wipe with disinfectant cleaning solution daily all wash rooms. This also includes all vertical partitions, dispensers, paper holders, sinks, faucets, and commodes.

- Wipe down all tables, chairs, and chair arms in public and meeting areas with disinfectant on a weekly basis.

- Clean all stairwell railings throughout the building on a weekly basis. Clean any stepwell railings within tenant spaces nightly.

- Spray all mats and elevator cab carpets weekly with an EPA-registered disinfectant.

- Clean all door release buttons and card readers daily.

- Clean and disinfect all drinking fountains daily.

- Clean and disinfect all push bars and push plates of all doors daily.

- If your building provides showers, they need to be cleaned and disinfected daily.

- Clean and disinfect the exterior of all microwaves and refrigerators daily.

- Clean and disinfect all table lamp knobs every Monday, Wednesday, and Friday.

- Sanitize all hard surfaces in food and coffee areas daily. This includes all tenant spaces.

Alert Level 5—The building implements the use of hand sanitizers by all building personnel, security officers, and cleaning employees as well as anyone entering the building. Cleaning specifications will depend upon the number of cleaning people available. A day porter or matron may be assigned for specific duties depending upon the size of the building. Continue the use of disposable latex gloves.

- Increase elevator cleaning to three times daily.

- Handles on both sides of all doors throughout the building will be wiped with disinfectant cleaning solution every other day.

- Clean all light switches and thermostats throughout the building daily.

- Increase the cleaning of wash rooms to twice daily.

- Wipe down all tables and chairs in public and meeting areas with disinfectant every Monday, Wednesday, and Friday.

- Increase the cleaning of stairwell railings throughout the building every Monday, Wednesday, and Friday. Wipe any stepwell railings within tenant spaces every evening.

- Spray all mats and elevator cab carpets every Monday, Wednesday, and Friday with an EPA-registered disinfectant.

- Increase the cleaning of door release buttons and card readers to 3 times daily.

- Clean and disinfect all drinking fountains three times per day.

- Clean and disinfect all push bars and push plates of all doors three times per day.

- Clean and disinfect exterior of all microwaves and refrigerators daily after morning rush and lunch rush.

- Clean and disinfect all table lamp knobs daily.

- Increase the cleaning of all hard surfaces in food and coffee areas prior to morning and lunch rushes.

Alert Level 6—This is the highest alert level and may require extreme measures contingent upon the nature and severity of the situation. The use of disposable gloves and masks will be required by all building personnel, security officers, and cleaning personnel wherever applicable.

The type and amount of cleaning will be determined by the management and approved by the owner. A day porter or matron may be assigned by the cleaning company for specific duties. Examples follow:

- Increase the cleaning of elevators to hourly.

- Increase the cleaning of doors to twice daily.

- Increase the cleaning of wash rooms to three times per day.

- Wipe down all tables and chairs in all public and meeting areas with disinfectant after every use, unless management has closed any or all of these areas.

- Clean all stairwell railings throughout the building every day. Clean any stepwell railings within tenant spaces three times per day.

- Spray all mats and elevator cab carpets every day with an EPA registered disinfectant.

- Clean all door release buttons and card readers every hour.

- Close off drinking fountains.

- Clean and disinfect all push bars and push plates of all doors every hour.

Emergency Cleanup Services

Influenza viruses may live on hard surfaces for up to two days. Remove viruses with a neutral detergent followed by a disinfectant solution. This includes any excrement.

In the event that employees have been evacuated from an affected area when an outbreak begins, special cleanup services will commence. These services will be performed by firms specialized in these services, hired by management and approved by the owner of the building.

Security Guidelines

Ongoing Personnel Training

As the threat of an influenza pandemic increases, heightened security is necessary. This includes cross-training to help minimize disruption and ensure continued service. If the building uses an outside contractor as opposed to on-site personnel, make sure your contract covers cross-training of its personnel; and that they have a response plan in place to ensure they are able to provide contracted services in the event that an influenza pandemic occurs.

The labor pool can be greatly reduced due to transportation, employee demographics, and level of panic in the community. Therefore, it is critical to have security officers, who live within a short distance, trained in the building's specifications, and the building's Post Orders.

- Post a written job description at the security officer's station of each officer's responsibilities relating to their respective shifts during a normal operation.

- Spell out the specific duties that will be carried out by each security officer through each level of influenza pandemic.

- Inform all security officers that there will be no hand shaking or any other physical contact with another person. They are also to use their arm to cover coughing or sneezing and avoid touching their eyes, nose, and mouth. Ensure that employees always wash their hands.

- If using contracted services, the contract supervisor will give management an up-to-date listing of each security officer working in the building and those cross trained. This listing will include their address, proximity to the building, and emergency telephone number.

Secure the Building

Alert Levels 1–4—The building acts in a normal operational mode. Security will be performed as normally contracted and in accordance with the building's post orders.

Alert Level 5—The building implements the use of hand sanitizers by all building staff, security officers, and cleaners. The use of disposable gloves and masks will also be required.

- Identify those tenants with special needs and incorporate those needs without jeopardizing the building's health and safety.

- In the event that tenants decide to restrict visitors, guests, and employees, they will inform the security officer.

Alert Level 6—The building will be placed in off-hours mode per the building's post orders. All persons will sign in at the security officer's desk.

Prevent Unauthorized Entry

Alert Levels 1–5—The building acts in a normal operational mode, contingent upon tenants deciding to restrict certain access of their employees and guests. Security will be performed as normally contracted and in accordance with the building's post orders.

Alert Level 6—The building implements the use of hand sanitizers by all building staff, security officers, and cleaning personnel. The use of disposable gloves and masks will also be required.

- All persons, including those with key cards, may be limited to a specific entrance. This will be determined by building management pending lease terms.

- All building personnel and building services vendors entering the building will be given disposable gloves and masks to wear while they are in the building. Upon exiting the building, they will dispose of the gloves and masks in a special bin.

- Visitor access may be limited to scheduled appointments only.

Enforce Hygiene upon Entering the Building

Alert Levels 1–4—The building acts in a normal operational mode.

Alert Level 5—The security officers shall make sure that all persons entering the building will clean their hands with sanitizer. The security officers will also remind everyone not to have any physical contact with other persons, including hand shaking. They are to also use their arms to cover any coughing or sneezing; and they should avoid touching their eyes, nose, and mouth.

Alert Level 6—The security officers shall make sure that all persons entering the building will clean their hands with sanitizer. Each building services vendor will be given a pair of latex gloves and a mask, which will be worn during their duration in the building. As these vendors exit the building, they will place the gloves and masks in a special bin. Security officers, cleaning personnel, and building personnel will wear latex gloves whenever handling any type of mail, newspapers, magazines, or when engaging in any other hand contact.

Banning of Foreign Travelers

Alert Levels 1–5—The building acts in a normal operational mode. Security will be performed as normally contracted and in accordance with the building's post orders pertaining to foreign travelers.

Alert Level 6—The building will be placed in off-hours mode twenty four hours per day. No building personnel or building services vendor will be allowed to enter if they have visited any countries impacted with influenza pandemic.

Building Maintenance Guidelines

HVAC Mechanical Operations—Because the flu is transmitted through droplets carrying the influenza virus, the building's heating, ventilation, and air conditioning are of major concern. Persons working on these systems must wear protective equipment whenever working in these areas and they must wash their hands often. Some guidelines follow.

- Increase the amount of outside air and reduce the amount of recirculated air.
- Increase the frequency at which air-handling device filters are changed.
- Use HEPA air filters to improve air quality.
- Check operation of all air handler units every day. Log and report any problems to HVAC service contractor.

These measures will depend on the type of HVAC systems.

Ordering of Critical Supplies

The following timelines are suggested prior to alert level 4 because there may not be any supplies available once Alert Levels 4–6 have been reached.

Alert Levels 1-2—Management will order safety supplies such as face masks and latex gloves. Ensure vendors have a three-month stock.

Alert Level 3—Management will order supplies from the following vendors:
(list at least three vendors with office, cell, and e-mail addresses)

The building uses the following supplies:

(list all supplies with specific details and from which vendor)

While the following products are suggested for cleaning during certain alert levels, it is good practice to check with a reliable source beforehand.

- Butchers Bright: A ready-to-use foaming product that can be used on all surfaces above the floor. It has a three-minute dwell time.

- Butchers Heptagon: A ready-to-use liquid product that can be used on all surfaces above the floor. It has a three-minute dwell time.

- Butchers Dimension: A concentrated product that needs to be mixed with water. This would be used for mopping floors and could also be put in a spray bottle for general cleaning. It has a ten-minute dwell time and is known to dry streak free.

Drinking Fountain Operations

Alert Levels 1–5—The building acts in a normal operational mode.

Alert Level 6—If drinking fountains are available in the building (including tenant spaces), building maintenance will shut them down and cover them in plastic. A note will be placed on top stating, "Shut down until further notice. Do not use!"

Managing Agent Guidelines

Service Providers

It is imperative that the service providers have their personnel cross-trained and retain an adequate stocking of necessary supplies. The managing agent will monitor the progress of these vendors throughout the different alert levels using a grid designed in accordance with the building's needs for such vendors.

Personnel Cross-Training

The number of personnel for cross-training will depend upon the size of the building. Cross-training of these positions is as follows.

- A job description of each employee's current duties will be posted on the bulletin board in the building maintenance office.

- Other employees, who live within fifteen miles of the building, will be trained in the job descriptions and should be familiar with the standard building operations. They will have a copy of the standard operating procedures manual at their disposal. The property manager and operations manager will confirm that these employees feel comfortable in their roles.

- Management will spell out the specific duties that will be carried out by each employee through each alert level of influenza pandemic.

- A listing of each person cross-trained in the job duties will be posted in the building maintenance office. The listing will include their address, proximity to the building, and emergency telephone number.

- The property manager and operations manager will determine when the cross-trained person will be engaged and what hours they will work.

In the event that the property manager or operations manager is not available to oversee the operations of the building, the managing director would assume these duties or assign them to another qualified individual. An organization chart can be found in the appendices.

Communications

Alert Levels 1–3—The building acts in a normal operational mode.

Alert Levels 4–6—The communications given to tenants will be determined by management through the owner and the local health department's directive.

- Management will instruct building maintenance to post a sign at all entrances to the building stating the following: "This building is using preventive measures to control influenza pandemic. Please use the pedestal sanitizer upon entering. You will find these placed throughout the building for your use at all times." Personnel should avoid hand shaking; and use a tissue or their arm to cover any coughing or sneezing. Also, they must avoid touching their eyes, nose, and mouth, as well as wash their hands frequently.

- Once the proper communication has been determined for the tenants, management will contact building maintenance. Building maintenance will then instruct the security officer to contact all emergency response coordinators of tenants via telephone or a prepared e-mail statement and advise them of then current local health department restrictions. These procedures are contingent upon the size of the building and its structure of building personnel.

- In the event that a communication needs to be given to the entire building, building maintenance will use the manual audio at the panel (if applicable in the building) to convey the following: "We wish to alert all tenants that the government has mandated the following .... Please proceed accordingly."

- In the event that media approaches any building personnel, security, or cleaning staff, state the following: "I don't know the particulars and don't want to give misinformation. Please contact ... at ... and he/she will be prepared to entertain your questions."

- An employee from management will have a desk on the first floor with telephone and computer to be a conduit for incoming and outgoing information. This will also be used for scheduling personnel, vendor information, and any other type of needed communication. He or she will monitor local news stations and websites for public transportation disruptions, quarantine request, medical facility availability, and more. This person will also contact state or local public health agencies to request current information on vaccine or antiviral availability and other flu control recommendations.

Employee Face-to-Face Guidelines

In the event that the building uses union employees, management needs to understand the impact of issues like union rules on these employees. The following is recommended contingent upon union rules, if applicable.

Alert Levels 1–3—The building acts in a normal operational mode; and all building personnel and building services vendors will practice the use of personal hygiene etiquette. Building maintenance will post a sign in all wash rooms stating the following: "Please wash your hands before leaving this area."

Alert Levels 4–5—While in the building, building personnel and building services vendors will not have any physical contact with other persons, including hand shaking. They will also be reminded to use their arms to cover any coughing or sneezing and to avoid touching their eyes, nose, and mouth.

Alert Level 6—All building personnel and building services vendors will wear latex gloves and masks while in the building. The building will recommend to the tenants that there will be no gatherings of large groups. Handling of any type of mail, newspapers, or magazines, or engaging in any other hand contact, requires wearing latex disposable gloves.

Food Sanitation Measures

Alert Levels 1–3—The building acts in a normal operational mode; and all building personnel and building services vendors will practice the use of personal hygiene etiquette.

Alert Levels 4–5—Management will ensure that all public food areas are supplied with only silverware, plates, cups, and glasses that are wrapped in plastic plus providing only food items that are individually packaged. No cutting boards will be provided.

Alert Level 6—A sign will be posted in all public food areas stating: "Please wipe your tray before and after use with the sanitizing wipes provided."

Tenant Responsibilities

As the alert levels heighten, tenants are responsible for their own protocols for their personnel and guests, contingent upon any government mandate. Management will remind tenants to have their employees frequently wash their hands.

Practice Drills

Tabletop Exercise—The exact timing and circumstances of an influenza pandemic won't be known until the event is upon us. A proactive effort is to have practice drills. One such drill is called a tabletop exercise. This involves the decision team discussing what action steps are in their plans. Examples of action steps include:

- Key personnel and service providers can be contacted quickly.
- Key personnel and service providers are aware of their duties.
- Cross-trainers are comfortable in their roles.
- All available resources are identified.
- All contingencies are accurate and complete.
- All necessary vital records are available.
- Employees and service providers are properly scheduled as alert levels rise.
- Personnel can perform tasks with back-up equipment or systems when normal communications and utilities are not functioning.

More examples can be found in the appendix entitled "Influenza Pandemic Outline for Building Operations."

Functional Exercise—This exercise would be used when the decision team actually performs the activities called for in their plans. They would be given a scenario where they go through the preparations for acting out an influenza pandemic.

Following each exercise, the decision team would discuss their observations and feedback. An after-action report would be given to management summarizing all observations and comments.

Decision Team—The decision team should include some or all of the following as applicable in each building: property manager, head of building maintenance, head of building operations, security supervisor, cleaning area manager, and any other key individuals that would add to the specific situation. Be prepared to have an alternate in the event that one or more of the team contracts the virus. On occasion a representative from the Center for Disease Control and Prevention or from a city health department may be invited to attend.

The decision team needs to consider that government agencies may discontinue providing non-vital services, medical services may be overwhelmed, the ability to diagnose influenza may be challenging, protective equipment such as surgical masks may be in short supply, public transportation may be limited or halted, and absenteeism among utility workers may impact repairs and customer services. These are just a few of a myriad of services that could be affected in an influenza pandemic; and the decision team needs to be prepared for these occurrences.

All members of the decision team need to be comfortable in their roles, understand their responsibilities, and be able to implement them (this is especially critical for the alternates).

Post-Influenza Pandemic

Staffing Duties—In the event that building maintenance had been infected with the influenza and cross-trained employees were substituted, the cross-trained employees will continue the work schedule until such time as building maintenance returns.

Site Safety and Security Duties—In the event that the property manager cannot notify the tenants directly, he or she will give a script for the security officers to notify all tenants that normal operations have been restored. The script will read: "Please be aware that normal operations in the building have been restored. However, if you discover anything out of the ordinary, please notify building maintenance." Building maintenance will ensure that all card readers, video surveillance, fire, and life safety monitoring capabilities are functioning properly.

Restoring Operations to Normal—Building maintenance will use the following guidelines for returning to normal operation.

- Evaluate the adjusting of air handling and ventilation systems.
- Validate that water, wastewater, and natural gas lines have not been damaged and are functioning properly.
- Have the cleaning company empty bins with disposable gloves and masks, as directed by the health department.
- Ensure all common areas and equipment have been thoroughly sanitized.
- Reinstate all operating functions that had been suspended.
- Restore all drinking fountains to their normal operation.
- Remove all signage relating to the influenza pandemic.

The property manager and operations manager will use the following guidelines for returning to normal operation.

- Inform the tenants of any new operating procedures that may impact them.
- Notify all service providers and suppliers when normal operations will be resumed.
- Inform personnel of the return to normal operations and of any new policies that have been or will be instituted.
- Offer and implement any type of support needed to alleviate any reluctance to enter the building.

Appendix

Cleaning Schedule Guidelines

Duty	Level Four	Level Five	Level Six
Elevator call buttons	Wash daily	Three times daily	Wash hourly
Desks, copiers, other equipment	Wipe daily	Wipe daily	Wipe daily, wash weekly
**Telephones	Spray daily	Spray daily	Spray daily
Door handles on both sides	Wash Mon.,Wed.,Fri.	Wash daily	Wash two times daily
Light switches	Wipe Mon.,Wed.,Fri.	Wipe daily	Wipe daily, wash weekly
Thermostats	Wipe Mon.,Wed.,Fri.	Wipe daily	Wipe daily, wash weekly
Wash rooms horizontal surfaces	Wash daily	Wash twice daily	Wash three times daily
Tables in public and meeting areas	Wipe weekly	Wipe Mon., Wed., Fri.	After every use unless shut down
Chairs in public and meeting areas	Wipe weekly	Wipe Mon., Wed., Fri.	After every use unless shut down
Stairwell railings	Wipe weekly	Wipe Mon., Wed., Fri.	Wipe daily, wash weekly
Stepwells within tenant spaces	Wipe nightly	Wipe once a day & night	Wipe three times daily
Mats and elevator cab carpets	Spray weekly	Spray Mon., Wed., Fri.	Spray daily
Door release buttons	Wash daily	Wash three times daily	Wipe every hour
Card readers	Wash daily	Wash three times daily	Wipe every hour
Drinking fountains	Wash daily	Wash three times daily	Closed, no need for cleaning
Push bars and push plates	Wash daily	Wash three times daily	Wipe every hour
Stall showers	Wash daily	Wash daily	Wash daily
Microwaves and refrigerators	Wash daily	After morning/afternoon rush	After morning/afternoon rush
Table lamp knobs	Wipe Mon., Wed.,Fri.	Wipe daily	Wipe daily

**It is each tenant's responsibility to have their personnel clean their own areas throughout the day.

Influenza Pandemic Outline for Building Operations Checklist

1. Define the building systems that are mission critical. _____
_____
_____
_____

2. Number man hours needed to support their operation. _____

3. Define the skills needed to support their operation. _____
_____
_____

4. Define what functions can be managed remotely. _____
_____

5. If none, can any be retrofitted and if yes, how much? _____

6. If the building would be closed due to epidemic, what
functions needed to shut down building systems? _____
_____
_____

7. List service providers, telephone numbers, locations,
addresses. _____
_____

8. List employees within those firms, telephone numbers,
cell telephone numbers, their home addresses. _____
_____

9. List critical supplies needed during a pandemic. _____
_____

10. List water coolers and how to shut them off. _____

Other Recommendations

1. Cross train employees.
2. If service providers or suppliers don't have alternate
sources, building needs to secure them.
3. Work with adjoining building to assist when needed.
4. Stockpile critical supplies.
5. Develop "how to" procedures for execution of
critical tasks.
6. Set up programs for operating off site.
7. Set up program for tenants to report to property manager
weekly once Alert Level 4 reached.
8. Plan for emergency clean-up services.
9. Possible relocating to temporary space.
10. Set up cleaning procedures at different levels of pandemic.
11. Set up building hygiene procedures at different levels of
pandemic.
12. Set up conduit for communications with tenants,
providers, and any other critical resouces.
13. Establish sick-tenant protocols.
14. What to do if need to quarantine entire floors.
15. Policy for denying access to those showing signs of illness.
16. At level 5 and 6 ban foreign travelers and packages.

Influenza Pandemic Organization Guide

Building Hours: _____

Days of Operations:

Full Time Personnel:

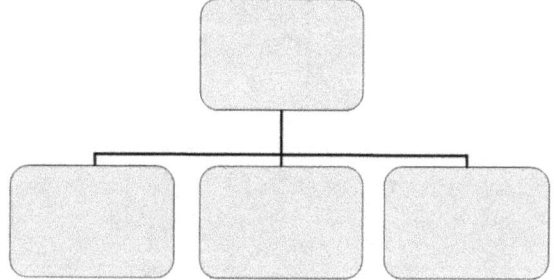

Cross-Trained Personnel:

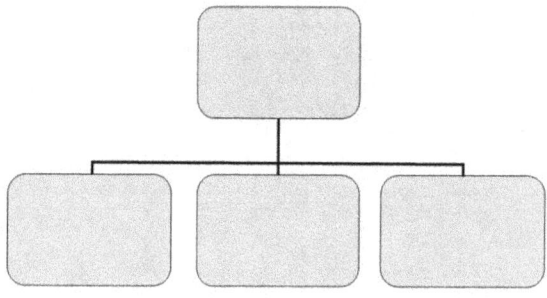

Summary

The material and information in this manual are designed to aid the reader in protecting his or her building as much as possible, and to provide for a healthier environment during an influenza pandemic. The charts and graphs are helpful tools, created to facilitate the flow of information.

Karen J. Bates

Karen retired as senior vice president of a very prestigious commercial real estate firm in 2007 and continues to work as a consultant in a range of commercial real estate companies. Throughout her 39 years of property management, she managed buildings as large as 700,000 square feet. One of her personal achievements was managing a winning campaign for a person running for a position in local government.